Basic Cuing for Pilates Teachers

by Laurette Ryan, PMA_CPT

a sincere dedication to the
inspirational teaching styles
of my favorite
1st Generation Pilates Teachers,
Ron Fletcher ,Kathy Grant
and Mary Bowen.
who have sparked
in so many the desire
to dig deeper an become ,
BE more through movement.

Contents

Introduction..........................1
Cuing Is................................3
Beginning class..................7
Verbal Cuing.....................13
Anatomical Cuing............21
Visualization Cuing.........25
Teacher Exercises...........35
Final Thoughts.................39

Introduction

The first movement class I ever taught was a series of dance classes when I was fifteen years old. It took place at my high school , the participants had never taken a class and were unaware of dance terminology and had no experience with the nature of the movements I wished to teach them.

Wanting at this time in my life, to impress my teacher with my wonderful skills as a dancer myself, this put the situation in an interesting light.

I knew what I wanted them to do, how it would look, what it would feel like- in my body......how do you get them- to do, to look, to feel? CUING.

Through that series of classes most of my cuing was demonstration. The I do- you copy method. I was frustrated a bit when I realized that I seem to lack the verbal skills necessary to verbally cue my class. I had participated for years in classes where the most wonderful teachers-never did any or very little of the dance and created beautiful movement. They made it look easy.

What I learned that semester was -it wasn't easy and if I was going to teach and be a good teacher – I had to figure this "cuing" thing out.

This book is created for those wishing to become better at communicating to their students – "the how" of movement. The "**how**" including what to do and what to feel and **how** to even expand that, in order for movement to be more than just the copycat experience. This book is designed for movement teachers and as such will focus on movements used in that modality.

Cuing is .....

There are different ways to cue movement. They are all ways of communicating what you want someone else's body to do.

No wonder this is difficult. There are times we can't even communicate to our own bodies what we want them to do.

The body, to do any movement, no matter how simple, processes thousands upon thousands of messages. Information , tons of information is relayed in and out of the system and then we -take a step....raise a hand....nod the head.

It really can be overwhelming, but you as teacher can make use of this wonderful complexity to give the student a more fulfilling experience in your class.

We are all multi-faceted communicators.
We communicate visually, verbally , kinesthetically and emotionally.

Visual communication is what we see. Demonstration teaching- I do....you copy .

Most times this style is very simplistic. Many times visual cuing produces movement which lacks motivation on a deeper level.

However if the teacher is very skilled and can incorporate tone, emotion and feeling into the visual, this can be very compelling. It requires, like all good teaching, an intimate connection with the student, a rapport.

When communicating verbally – there are many aspects to be considered .

What is said. How it is said or "tone". How many times is it said. Basically the verbal cuing – what you say can be broken into two parts.

The first is how to position the body to begin and the second part is telling the student what movement you want to achieve.

Having accomplished this – verbal cuing should ideally impart even more as to affect the feel and impact of the movement.

Kinesthetic communication is all about the feel, the touch , the sensation.

From the external this means
I tell you soften your shoulders-
then touch your shoulders-
you respond....
by softening the shoulders.

This communication is quick and effective the body does not need to process the words... as much.

Kinesthetic cuing additionally asks the student to experience on a deeper level the movement , to notice what it feels like.

Emotionally, the body on the deepest level is always present always reacting. The ultimate goal is to bring an awareness to the surface through the verbal, visual and kinesthetic technique.

The fully integrated and present body gets the best work done. If cuing/communicating touches this level, the student has a fulfilling experience and the teacher truly teaches the body.

When new to teaching you too, may start out with the I do-you copy method or demonstration teaching/instruction.

Soon however you need to really "teach" your work. What you need to begin doing this is to be able to say it- so they can do it. So let's start at the beginning to sharpen your verbiage.

That is - What do I call it? How do I say it?

Beginning the Class

To cue the participants in a standing position, you will decide whether you will cue from the feet up or the head down.

If starting at the feet one may say feet are in Pilates stance or parallel .

Describe how the feet are in contact with the floor...weight even in the toes and heels, all ten toes feeling the floor or mat.

Next move up the leg , knees aligned with the second and third toe of the foot , the muscles of the thighs...
inner thighs connected in the turned out at hip/ Pilates stance position.

Then to hip placement- hip bones(asis) pointing straight ahead, front hip bones and pubic bone level in the frontal plane.

Belly button/navel pulled in towards the spine , create length between the hips and ribs, front of the ribs lined up with the hip bones to the front.

Scapular/shoulder blades flat on the back, shoulders aligned under the ears, arms at the sides, inside of elbows facing front, neck lengthened, crown of the head reaching to the sky .

Additionally you can cue tail bone to the ground, breathing into the back of the rib cage.

Beginning cues on the breathing are themselves, most beneficial to set the tone for the class. Breath puts us in touch with that deeper level in our bodies as well as is a primary facilitator of all movement to follow.

Additionally, (you may not use all of these every time) many times you will want to say it as simply as possible.

An Example :
        Instead of-
" move your pelvis so that the the bones you feel on the front which are your hip bones and your pubic bone line up flat in front so that no one bone sticks out further than any other"
        you can say:
"hip bones and pubic bone -flat in the frontal plane"
Keeping the anatomical cuing down to a minimum –leaves more time to expand on the kinesthetic and emotional aspects.

Saying what to do, where everything goes is your first job ,but then saying how to do it – how meaning the feeling the tone and the emotion is the key to great cuing.

Generally from standing we need to get students on to the mat....say have a seat – at the end of your mat .... or stand at the end of your mat , cross your legs and sit down......or stand at the end facing your mat and roll down till your hands touch the floor, walk your hands out to plank.....make it simple – because it is.

Transitioning to Lying on the Back Supine

To lie on the back from seated- roll down vertebrae by vertebrae till you are lying flat on the mat...

Where are your feet? .....feet lined up with the sitz bones, knees bent

Where are your arms ? Arms by your sides, fingers reaching toward the end of your mat (toward your feet/ toward your toes)

Scapular or shoulder blades slide down the back.....

Where is your head? Lengthen the back of the neck by tucking the chin slightly..

Body in position......describe the breathing.....

Breath sweet breath

Breathing facilitates movement, it moves the movement and is a primary factor in Pilates work. The breath is felt through every part of the body.

We use the breath to bring the muscles deeper into contraction or remind the connective tissues of their length . We breath deeply into the basement of the lungs for the deep connection and foundation to breath.

Breathe into the back of the rib cage...the lungs are there!

Let the ribs to the back expand like a giant bellows. Feel the ribs spread like opening your fingers from a closed hand to one which is with fingers spread wide.

When lying on the back...as you breath into the back of the rib cage, feel the ribs behind you imprint on to the mat , pressing gently downward as if you were lying in sand on a beach making the ribs imprint behind you.

Feel the breath like you are filling a bucket of water – fill the lungs from the bottom to the top and empty the bucket /(your lungs) from the top to the bottom.

Check your breath to be smooth, with no rough edges, no jagged edges. Feel the breath at the back of the throat. Take time feel the breath...in the spine, at the sacrum , through the hip..... where else?

Verbal Cuing

Example:

Roll-up

the body start position- lying on your back,

the anatomical movement- raise arms up to ceiling, bring the armpits to the hips, lift the head, shoulders and scapular, peel the vertebra one at a time off the mat to come to a seated position, then roll back down, vertebra by vertebra till you are lying back.

Example:

Single Knee stretch

thebody start position- Lie on your back , knees in chair position, lift head , shoulders, scapular or come up to your c-curve , fingertips on the knees (or more advanced specific placement)

the anatomical movement- extend one leg out on a diagonal and then change, keeps your hips still. Reach for the opposite wall/ or where the wall and ceiling meet.

Example:

Double knee stretch

the body start position – lie on your back, knees in chair, c-curve, lift the head, shoulders and scapular, fingertips on the knees

the anatomical movement - both legs extend out to opposite wall , both arms extend over head, biceps by the ears and then arms and legs return to start position

For every exercise, the verbal cuing consists of two parts; the body start position and the anatomical movement cue. The body start position is the position of the body prior to any movement.

There are a few key positions and several variations of the basics. We will explore the simplest ways to get the body into position - verbally.

The anatomical movement cue is slightly more complex, but we will find ways to say what you want in the most direct and effective way.

Supine- to lie on your back.....

We could say take the supine position, of course, most students would have no idea what you meant ; so we say....lie on your back....

from here you must say where you want arms .legs and head....

Arms can be :

by your sides
in close to your body,
reaching or soft
by the sides on the floor, or slightly raised
reaching to the ceiling or at various angles...

Legs can be:

straight on the floor
knees bent, feet lined up with sitz bones on the mat
together
apart in parallel
knees in chair/ tabletop
legs up to the ceiling or at an angle
one leg or two legs in a particular position

Head can be:

resting on the floor
lifted (as in head shoulders scapular off the floor)
(c-curve)

In the supine position –

say where each thing (arms, legs, head)
 should be- in one cue for each.....
if the student doesn't respond with the appropriate action , --only then say it another way...or demonstrate.

Simple is best....for supine leg circles- say ....lie on your back , arms by your sides, right leg up to the ceiling, left leg down the mat....

note: I did not add a cue for head because it is probably where I already need it....on the floor...don't waste words -telling them to do ,what is already anatomically done. Now we can describe movement........

Side Lying:

to get here say: lie on your side (you knew that)
to align the spine you could say; line up your back with
the back edge of your mat, stack- hip over hip,

Where is your head? Are the legs straight, slightly bent, at
what angle from the hip?
Allow yourself only two to four anatomical cues after- lie
on your side- to relay the most important information.

In side lying I need to know where are my legs , head and
what is my spine/abs doing?

Prone:
to take the student prone---- you can if you've taught them say "prone position "and there they go....

You can say "prone position, on your tummies" now you've taught the ones who were listening – what prone position is.....and then next time if you just say prone position...they will go and the others *may* follow.

Say: lie on your stomach, lie on your belly/tummy,
     lie face down.

From here :
where are the legs? Together, apart....
Where is the upper body? Are they flat – say lie flat, head to one side or lace fingers -forehead on hands, or is the upper body raised?

Are we "propped on the elbows" like modified swan/cobra or raised up the hands -full swan/cobra style. With the upper body raised – cue shoulders blades down the back or away from the ears..

Where is the spine or abs? Abs in, spine long , no lumbar pressure. Where is the head? Looking up, straight , down?

And finally seated:
say: sit on your mat………. now….

Where are the legs? Together to the front, in a straddle, feet parallel or turned out, soles together (as in cobbler stretch or butterfly) legs to the side (as in mermaid or side bend) both legs or one……

Where are the arms?

The head? If necessary………

The spine/ abs?

The major body start positions are, standing, supine, side-lying, prone and seated, additionally kneeling and all fours. The positions are easy to cue by merely saying which position you want and then saying where the legs, arms, and sometimes, head, spine,(if not already there) need to be.

Now you can begin the second part of the cuing …the movement….

Anatomical Cuing

There are many ways to cue a movement , many words to describe the action you wish to instruct.

In the beginning using the simplest words is most effective. As you progress, and your desire should be to impart more than just "what " to do – but of course "how" to do it,...your words can be more colorful and precise.

By example we can say - "lift" the leg or "raise " the leg...but to give more information we could say....... float the leg, shoot the leg up, push the leg, reach the leg to......these are just a start.

Shoot the leg up and float the leg obviously accomplish the same lifting of the leg but with a very different pace , tone and intensity.

Below is a list of descriptive movement words. Included are many, but you could brainstorm more.

Movement Words
(the ones in bold we use the most)

raise, lift, float, shoot, push, throw, heave, elevate, reach, fly, soar, give energy to.

extend, elongate, lengthen, stretch, unfurl, draw out, open, increase, unfold, unroll, fan out, grow.

lower, descend, depress, release, sink, submerge, droop, drop.

curl, roll, wind, unwind, twist, twirl, curve, coil, bend, fold, bend, **flex.**

tighten, snake, uncoil, tilt, circle , arch, straighten,

contract, squeeze, clench, engage, hug, connect, activate. slither, relax, surrender, soften, fall, recede, climb, swoop, flutter, glide, slide, slip, let go of, melt. notice, become aware, smooth, feel, realize, untangle, unravel, flow.

The words previously noted are some to get your creative juices flowing.

Next try this exercise to see how you can begin to apply using creative, innovative effective language to get the results you want from your students.

Teacher Exercise:
Take some basic exercises you always use. Like the roll-up , the leg circle, spine twist – now write out a new movement cue to direct the student .

Such as:

Roll-up vertebrae by vertebrae and then roll away *uncoiling* the spine to the floor............

Add these and your own "juicy" words to your cuing and you begin to develop a style and a flavor to your classes and lessons.

Visualization Cuing

Creating Powerful Feeling Cues

To create a smooth and satisfying movement class, first you provide the frame or framework with good,solid -body and anatomical cuing. Now the student can do the exercise.

Next by offering a visualization you can help the student deeply connect to "the how" to do it.
 You involve the mind , the creative mind and not just the brain. Creating rich conceptual images during your cuing will enhance the students understanding and experience of the exercises you teach.

The physical brain decodes language and prompts the physical body to produce an action.

The mind however works on various levels simultaneously to produce a result in the physical, intellectual , emotional and yes even spiritual level of the student.

The mind is not only located in the brain, as in consciousness , but also is active in every cell of the body.

The body has a consciousness throughout, through and through at the cellular level and more.

When teaching, speaking with the student , not only is the brain decoding, but also the body is listening.

The body listens for the "feeling" cues. If the body is given very little or no feeling cues and or visualizations it can tune out... no information there to process.

It can rely on the directions given to it by the brain and move in a fairly mechanical matter.

We all have seen instances where we are asked to do something and maybe we are adverse to it or indifferent- we do the job , but it is hardly ever our best effort or result.

However when we are whole-heartedly, body mind and soul engaged in an effort , the results are always superior and far more fulfilling.

So then how do we get our students and ourselves to access that superior and more fulfilling experience?

We must create an emotional awareness, a intellectual engagement, a cognizant desire to fully commit to the activity, movement or exercise.

We do this with visualization .

Try this.

Relax the biceps in your arms.
Fairly easy, you feel the arms relax.

But what if you imagine :

your biceps being stroked by the softest lambs wool which releases any and all tension from the front of your shoulder to the inside of your elbow.

There is significant difference in the depth of the physical reaction and the commitment and awareness to the action.

Most student can read how to do an exercise, copy an exercise tape or just do what someone taught them long ago.

It is the responsibility of the teacher to make the lesson, workout or class, more than going through the motions.

To imprint the body with a new experience, to create a new and desirable pattern.

The potential of most bodies is never fully realized ,old limiting patterns and messages are all that ever get presented to the system.

The brain sees limits, the mind knows none. Inspiring the "mind" of the body, creates more fantastic results, than telling the brain what to do, ever will.

I believe anyone with a strong desire to teach, can learn to use and create powerful cues by getting in touch with your own sense of emotionally and kinesthetically what is happening in your own body during movement .

Watch the world around you and relate that to the movements and experience in your own physical presence.

It is often said that Pilates and other movement modalities are difficult to teach **well,** unless you've experienced them,.... done them "right"......and also for a period of time, so as they have imprinted themselves on your physical body.

This is important, because only then can you begin to bring in your experience of experiences in the world and in your body and relate them to someone else's.

In order to spark your own creativity, I will present to you some of my favorite visualizations. Some of which I am sure I have heard from someone else.

This is how it goes, and now you may take what I have to offer- use it as is, or expand upon it and take it in a whole new direction. My hope is that after trying on some of these your imagination erupts like a volcano, spewing out many more metaphors, feeling cues and visualizations than I have ever thought of, like tons and tons of molten lava -unstoppable.... wouldn't that be wonderful.

1) Imagine your head like a balloon full of air floating upward to the sky, lengthening the neck and spine creating stretched out spaces between the vertebrae. Feel how light the head is.

2) Feel the base of the neck rooted between the shoulder blades, feel the shoulder blades holding hands.

3) Allow your shoulders and shoulder blades to melt down your back like dripping candle wax.

4) Release the point between the head and neck, and gently balance the head over the sitz bones if sitting or feet if standing .

5) Drink in the air

6) Imagine you have air tanks strapped to your breath like a deep sea diver draw the breath in and out of the back of the ribcage where your air tanks are.

7) Your ribs are like an accordion expanding on the inhalation, squeezing out the air on exhalation.

8) Draw the breath down your spine like it is a hollow tube, follow it down and then up. Let it release the spine and fill the sacrum, expanding , weighting and releasing the back of the hips.

9) Spread the imaginary wings on your back with the inhalation, let them float back down on the exhale

10) Allow your shoulders to let go of your arms, your hips let go of your legs

11) To lengthen cervical spine, no wrinkles in the back of the neck.

12) Bring the armpits to the hips for shoulder stabilization, connect the lats and triceps with a fine thread or spiderweb, keep the spiderweb or thread in one piece, unbroken

13) Grow roots out of your heels and sacrum in standing, out of sacrum/sitz bones in seated position.

14) Lying supine, imagine the weight of your organs lying on the inside part of your spine.

15) Lying supine, imagine a lead apron draped over the front of you feel it weight you to the floor sinking the navel to the spine.

16) 16)Feel connection at various point through the body by the imagery of rubber bands or bungee cords connecting two points as in the sternum to the pubis or across hip bone to hip bone .

17) Use buttons or buttoning up metaphors to connect points

18) Get longer by growing as in a plant

19) To slow down in order to connect to as in realize, and imprint correct movement, imagine moving through jello, honey, soft clay.

20) In the prone position keep abdominals in by imagining a marble held in the navel, or keeping the belly away from the clothing as if a seamstresses pin was stuck in the shirt at the navel, or as if you were being tickled.

21) In supine imagine pelvis, sacrum , spine, ribs joints dissolving into the mat like water flowing into the floor

22) In standing let each of the toes feel the floor like fingers sinking into bread dough or pie crust.

23) In twisting the spine, imagine it as a spiral staircase

24) Feel a wide belt around the waist , cinch it in to a smaller circumference as in pull the belt tighter...

25) Imagine to hands one on the belly one on the low back, draw them together through the body as in prayer position.

This is a just a small sample of ideas for enticing the mind of the body to participate .

Images should be ones that most students can relate to.

Images of water, flying, floating, properties of sand, clay, heat or cold are things we can all imagine.

If the student can produce a kinesthetic image in the body's mind , they can create powerful deep movements on the physical level.

Teacher Exercises

To Develop Cuing Proficiency and Cultivate Creativity:

Exercise 1:

Divide your class format into several distinct segments.

Such as:

1. Standing Alignment,

2. Supine exercises, Seated exercises,

3. Side-lying Exercises,

4. Prone Exercises,

5. Class ending.

You may have more or less divisions but it is important to begin with a framework. Take each segment and one at a time , perhaps one per week, work to perfect the verbiage, words you'll use to improve that segment.

Breaking the class into segments allows you the time and framework of just a few exercises- to really improve your skills.

You can experiment a little and see what works without changing your whole class which is daunting and may not work or connect with your students the first time you try.

Additionally getting more creative with your cuing requires you to commit a little more emotionally , to become more vulnerable in your teaching. Like any new relationship (and this is developing a more intimate relationship with your students-make no doubt about it) your comfort level is paramount to your success.

EXERCISE 2:

You need several volunteers to get the most out of this exercise. Have your volunteers/students face the opposite direction from you or close their eyes.

You stay still and verbally teach an exercise. See how well they can follow your instruction. What can you do to improve your communication?

EXERCISE 3:

You need several students and one volunteer to provide feedback. Write a short list of exercises, which can only be seen by you and your feedback volunteer.

You will face away from the students , your feedback volunteer watches the class and can see which exercise you are trying to teach.

You verbally teach the exercise , your feedback volunteer lets you know whether your students are "getting it" .

What can you do to improve your skills?

FINAL THOUGHTS

Your desire to teach movement is a deep personal one.

Most teachers derive gratification and a sense of personal accomplishment from a well taught class.
We may enjoy financial rewards and social acclaim, but a far more powerful motivation is the joy we feel when our students "get it".

When they enjoy good health, body awareness, success in accomplishing new things and overall well-being.

When we excite and entice another human being to advance their quality of life.

If YOU can be an inspiration- YOU leave this world a better place.

And no contribution to that end is ever a small one.
So if you choose to teach- Teach the best you possibly can!
-Laurette Ryan

NOTES:

Made in the USA
San Bernardino, CA
11 October 2017